PELVIC FLOOR EXERCISES FOR SENIORS

Mastering Pelvic Floor Exercises For Vibrant Living With Pelvic Floor Exercises And Vaginal Training For Seniors

CONTENT

1: Introduction

2: The Basics of Pelvic Floor Health

3: Benefits of Pelvic Floor Exercises

4: Getting Started with Pelvic Floor Exercises

5: Pelvic Floor Exercise Techniques

6: Vaginal Training and Devices

7: Relaxation Techniques for Pelvic Floor Health

8: Addressing Incontinence

9: Managing Constipation

10: Healing Pelvic Pain

11: Creating a Sustainable Exercise Routine

12: Case Studies and Success Stories

13: Conclusion

INTRODUCTION

A. Purpose of the Book:

As we age, maintaining our health and independence becomes increasingly important. "Pelvic Floor Exercises for Seniors" is dedicated to empowering older adults with the knowledge and tools to improve their pelvic floor health. The purpose of this book is to provide a comprehensive guide to understanding and enhancing the function of the pelvic floor through simple, effective exercises tailored specifically for seniors.

B. Importance of Pelvic Floor Health in Seniors:

Pelvic floor health is a crucial aspect of overall well-being, particularly for seniors. The pelvic floor muscles support vital organs, including the bladder, intestines, and, in women, the uterus. These muscles play a significant role in controlling bladder and bowel functions, and their health directly impacts our quality of life. As we age, the pelvic floor can weaken, leading to issues such as incontinence, constipation, and pelvic pain. By prioritizing pelvic floor health, seniors can enjoy a higher quality of life, enhanced mobility, and greater independence.

C. Overview of Issues Addressed:

Incontinence, constipation, and pelvic pain are common issues that can significantly affect the lives of seniors. This book addresses these problems by offering non-surgical, exercise-based interventions designed to strengthen the pelvic floor muscles. Each chapter is crafted to provide practical solutions and routines that can be easily integrated into daily life, helping to alleviate symptoms and improve overall pelvic health.

D. Benefits of Non-Surgical Interventions:

Non-surgical interventions, such as pelvic floor exercises, offer numerous benefits. They are low-risk, cost-effective, and can be done in the comfort of one's home. These exercises not only strengthen the pelvic floor muscles but also improve core stability, enhance bladder and bowel control, and reduce pelvic pain. By following the guidance in this book, seniors can take proactive steps towards better pelvic health without the need for invasive procedures.

E. Understanding the Pelvic Floor:

To effectively engage in pelvic floor exercises, it's important to first understand the anatomy and function of this crucial muscle group.

F. Anatomy and Function of the Pelvic Floor:

The pelvic floor is a group of muscles and connective tissues that span the bottom of the pelvis, forming a supportive hammock for the pelvic organs. These muscles are responsible for maintaining continence, supporting pelvic organs, and contributing to sexual function. They play a vital role in everyday activities, such as walking, lifting, and even breathing.

G. Changes in the Pelvic Floor with Aging:

Aging brings about several changes in the body, and the pelvic floor is no exception. Hormonal changes, decreased muscle mass, and reduced collagen can lead to a weakening of the pelvic floor muscles. This weakening can result in a range of issues, from mild discomfort to significant health challenges. Understanding these changes is the first step towards addressing and mitigating their effects.

H. Common Problems Affecting the Pelvic Floor in Seniors:

Seniors often face specific pelvic floor issues, including urinary incontinence, fecal incontinence, constipation, and pelvic organ prolapse. These conditions can be distressing and impact daily activities and overall quality of life. This book delves into each of these problems, offering insights into their causes, symptoms, and most importantly, exercises that can help manage and improve these conditions.

"Pelvic Floor Exercises for Seniors" is more than just a guide; it is a companion on your journey to better health. By understanding and caring for your pelvic floor, you can enjoy a more active, comfortable, and independent life. Let this book be your resource for achieving and maintaining optimal pelvic floor health.

THE BASICS OF PELVIC FLOOR HEALTH

A. What is the Pelvic Floor?

The pelvic floor is a crucial, yet often overlooked, component of the human body. It consists of a group of muscles, ligaments, and connective tissues that form a supportive hammock-like structure at the base of the pelvis. This structure spans the area from the pubic bone at the front to the tailbone at the back, encompassing the pelvic organs and playing a vital role in maintaining their proper function.

I. Muscles, Ligaments, and Connective Tissue:

The pelvic floor is composed of several key muscles, including the levator ani group (which includes the pubococcygeus, puborectalis, and iliococcygeus muscles) and the coccygeus muscle. These muscles are essential for various bodily functions, from supporting the pelvic organs to controlling the passage of urine and feces.

Levator Ani Group: This is the primary muscle group of the pelvic floor. The pubococcygeus muscle is particularly important as it wraps around the vagina in women and the prostate in men, providing essential support. The puborectalis muscle plays a crucial role in maintaining continence by forming a sling around the rectum, while the iliococcygeus muscle contributes to overall pelvic stability.

Coccygeus Muscle: This muscle assists the levator ani group in supporting the pelvic organs and stabilizing the pelvis.

Connective Tissues and Ligaments: The pelvic floor is further supported by various ligaments and connective tissues, including the endopelvic fascia and the uterosacral and cardinal ligaments. These structures help anchor the pelvic organs in place, ensuring they remain properly positioned.

II. Role in Supporting Pelvic Organs:

The pelvic floor's primary function is to support the pelvic organs, which include the bladder, uterus (in women), prostate (in men), and rectum. This support is essential for maintaining the proper alignment and function of these organs, preventing issues such as prolapse and incontinence.

Bladder: The pelvic floor muscles help control the release of urine by maintaining proper closure of the urethra.

Uterus and Vagina (in women): The pelvic floor provides critical support for the uterus and helps maintain vaginal tone and function.

Prostate (in men): The pelvic floor supports the prostate, which is essential for urinary and reproductive health.

Rectum: By forming a sling around the rectum, the pelvic floor muscles help maintain continence and support the rectal walls.

B. Common Pelvic Floor Disorders:

Despite its vital role, the pelvic floor can be prone to various disorders, especially as individuals age. Understanding these common issues is the first step toward effective management and treatment.

I. Types of Incontinence:

Incontinence is a prevalent issue among seniors, significantly impacting quality of life. There are three primary types of incontinence related to pelvic floor dysfunction:

Stress Incontinence: This occurs when physical activities such as coughing, sneezing, or lifting put pressure on the bladder, leading to involuntary urine leakage. Weak pelvic floor muscles are often the culprit.

Urge Incontinence: Also known as overactive bladder, this type is characterized by a sudden, intense urge to urinate, followed by involuntary urine leakage. It can be caused by nerve damage or muscle overactivity.

Mixed Incontinence: This is a combination of stress and urge incontinence, presenting symptoms of both conditions.

II. Pelvic Organ Prolapse:

Pelvic organ prolapse occurs when the pelvic organs descend from their normal position due to weakened pelvic floor muscles and connective tissues. This can lead to discomfort, pressure, and functional issues. Types of prolapse include:

Cystocele: Prolapse of the bladder into the vaginal wall.

Rectocele: Prolapse of the rectum into the vaginal wall.

Uterine Prolapse: Descent of the uterus into the vaginal canal.

III. Chronic Pelvic Pain:

Chronic pelvic pain is a persistent pain in the pelvic region that lasts for six months or more. This condition can significantly affect daily life and may be caused by various factors, including pelvic floor muscle dysfunction, inflammation, or nerve entrapment.

Muscle Dysfunction: Tension or spasms in the pelvic floor muscles can cause chronic pain.

Inflammation: Conditions such as interstitial cystitis can lead to chronic inflammation and pain in the pelvic region.

Nerve Entrapment: Nerves in the pelvic area, such as the pudendal nerve, can become compressed or irritated, leading to chronic pain.

IV. Constipation:

Constipation is another common issue that can be linked to pelvic floor dysfunction. It involves difficulty in passing stools and infrequent bowel movements. Pelvic floor disorders can contribute to constipation by impairing the coordination and strength needed for effective bowel movements.

Dyssynergic Defecation: This condition occurs when there is a lack of coordination between the pelvic floor muscles and the abdominal muscles during bowel movements.

Rectal Prolapse:NThe descent of the rectum can lead to difficulties in stool passage and contribute to constipation.

Understanding these common pelvic floor disorders highlights the importance of maintaining pelvic floor health, particularly as we age. In the next chapter, we will explore specific exercises designed to strengthen and support the pelvic floor, providing practical strategies for improving and maintaining pelvic health in seniors.

BENEFITS OF PELVIC FLOOR EXERCISES

Pelvic floor exercises, often known as Kegel exercises, have gained recognition for their significant health benefits, particularly for seniors. As we age, maintaining muscle strength and function becomes increasingly vital. This chapter will delve into the specific advantages of incorporating pelvic floor exercises into daily routines, highlighting their role in strengthening the pelvic floor and providing holistic health benefits.

A. Strengthening the Pelvic Floor:

I. How Exercises Improve Muscle Tone and Function:

The pelvic floor is a group of muscles that support the bladder, bowel, and, in women, the uterus. These muscles play a crucial role in controlling urination, bowel movements, and sexual function. Over time, factors such as aging, childbirth, and surgery can weaken the pelvic floor, leading to a host of issues. Pelvic floor exercises work by repeatedly contracting and relaxing these muscles, much like lifting weights strengthens arm muscles.

Regular practice of these exercises enhances muscle tone and function by:

Increasing Muscle Strength: Just like any other muscle group, the pelvic floor muscles grow stronger with regular exercise. Strengthening these muscles can help improve their ability to support pelvic organs and maintain proper function.

Improving Muscle Coordination: Pelvic floor exercises help train the muscles to contract and relax on demand, enhancing coordination and control. This is crucial for managing bladder and bowel functions.

Enhancing Blood Flow: Exercise promotes increased blood flow to the muscles, which is essential for muscle health and repair. Improved circulation helps maintain the elasticity and strength of the pelvic floor muscles.

II. Preventive Benefits Against Pelvic Floor Disorders:

Strong pelvic floor muscles can significantly reduce the risk of developing pelvic floor disorders, which are common in seniors. These disorders include urinary incontinence, fecal incontinence, and pelvic organ prolapse. Here's how pelvic floor exercises can act as a preventive measure:

Urinary Incontinence: Strengthening the pelvic floor muscles can help prevent stress incontinence (leakage of urine during activities that put pressure on the bladder, such as coughing or lifting) and urge incontinence (a sudden, intense urge to urinate).

Fecal Incontinence: By enhancing the strength and control of the pelvic floor muscles, individuals can better manage bowel movements, reducing the risk of accidental leakage.

Pelvic Organ Prolapse: This condition occurs when pelvic organs drop from their normal position due to weakened pelvic floor muscles.

Regular pelvic floor exercises can help maintain the muscles' strength, providing better support to the organs and reducing the risk of prolapse.

B. Holistic Health Benefits:

Beyond strengthening the pelvic floor, these exercises offer numerous holistic health benefits that contribute to overall well-being.

I. Enhanced Bladder and Bowel Control:

One of the most immediate and noticeable benefits of pelvic floor exercises is improved control over bladder and bowel functions. This improvement can lead to:

Increased Confidence: Knowing that one has better control over these essential bodily functions can greatly enhance self-esteem and reduce anxiety, particularly in social situations.

Reduced Frequency of Accidents: With stronger and more responsive pelvic floor muscles, the likelihood of accidental leakage is minimized, allowing for a more active and worry-free lifestyle.

Better Management of Chronic Conditions: For seniors managing conditions such as overactive bladder or irritable bowel syndrome, pelvic floor exercises can provide significant relief by improving muscle function and control.

II. Improved Sexual Health:

Pelvic floor health is closely linked to sexual health. Strengthening these muscles can lead to:

Enhanced Sexual Function: For both men and women, stronger pelvic floor muscles can enhance sexual pleasure by improving the ability to contract and control these muscles during sexual activity.

Increased Sensation: Improved muscle tone can lead to increased sensitivity and enjoyment during intercourse.

Reduced Pain: For women, strong pelvic floor muscles can help reduce discomfort or pain during intercourse, which can be a common issue as vaginal tissues change with age.

III. Reduced Risk of Surgery:

Maintaining a healthy pelvic floor can also reduce the likelihood of needing surgical interventions for pelvic floor disorders. Here's how:

Preventing the Need for Corrective Surgery: By strengthening the pelvic floor muscles, individuals can often manage or prevent the progression of conditions that might otherwise require surgical correction, such as severe pelvic organ prolapse.

Post-Surgery Recovery: For those who have undergone pelvic surgery, regular pelvic floor exercises can aid in recovery by enhancing muscle strength and function, thereby improving the overall outcome of the surgery.

GETTING STARTED WITH PELVIC FLOOR EXERCISES

A. Consulting with Healthcare Providers:

I. Importance of Professional Guidance:

Embarking on a journey to strengthen your pelvic floor muscles is a positive step toward enhancing your overall health and well-being. However, it's crucial to begin this journey with the right guidance. Consulting with healthcare providers, such as your primary care physician, a gynecologist, urologist, or a specialized physiotherapist, can provide invaluable insight into your specific needs and help tailor a program that's right for you.

Healthcare professionals can offer:

1. Personalized Assessment: They can assess your current pelvic floor condition and identify any underlying issues that may need to be addressed before starting exercises. This is particularly important for seniors who may

have specific medical conditions such as prolapse, incontinence, or post-surgical concerns.

2. Customized Exercise Plans: Based on your assessment, healthcare providers can recommend specific exercises that are safe and effective for your condition. They can guide you on the correct techniques and ensure you perform them correctly to avoid injury.

3. Monitoring Progress: Regular check-ins with your healthcare provider can help track your progress, make necessary adjustments to your exercise routine, and address any concerns or complications that may arise.

4. Support and Motivation: Having professional support can boost your confidence and keep you motivated, knowing you have a trusted expert to turn to with questions or issues.

II. Identifying the Right Exercises for Individual Needs:

Every individual has unique pelvic health needs, which is why a one-size-fits-all approach doesn't work. Your healthcare provider can help identify the exercises that will be most beneficial for you based on your specific conditions and goals.

For example:

For Incontinence: Specific exercises like Kegels can help strengthen the muscles that control urination.

on lifting and holding can help manage symptoms and prevent worsening of the condition.

Post-Surgery Recovery: After surgeries, such as prostatectomy or hysterectomy, tailored exercises can aid in recovery and restore pelvic floor strength.

By working with a healthcare provider, you can ensure that you are engaging in exercises that are not only effective but also safe for your particular situation.

B. Learning to Locate and Activate the Pelvic Floor Muscles:

I. Techniques for Finding the Right Muscles:

Before you can start strengthening your pelvic floor muscles, you need to know how to locate and activate them correctly. Here are some techniques to help you find the right muscles:

1. Stop the Flow: One common method to identify your pelvic floor muscles is to try and stop the flow of urine when you're in the middle of urinating. The muscles you use to do this are your pelvic floor muscles. However, it's important not to make a habit of stopping your urine flow regularly, as this can cause other issues.

2. Tighten and Lift: Imagine that you are trying to avoid passing gas. The muscles you

squeeze to prevent gas from escaping are your pelvic floor muscles. Similarly, imagine pulling these muscles up and inward, as if you are lifting something inside your pelvis.

3. Visual Aids: Using diagrams or models provided by your healthcare provider can also be beneficial. Visualizing the anatomy of the pelvic floor can help you better understand where these muscles are and how they function.

4. Biofeedback Devices: In some cases, your healthcare provider may recommend biofeedback devices that provide real-time feedback on muscle activation, helping you learn to control and strengthen these muscles more effectively.

II. Basic Exercises to Start With:

Once you've identified your pelvic floor muscles, you can begin with some basic exercises to start building strength and endurance. Here are a few beginner exercises to help you get started:

1. Basic Kegels:

Sit or lie down comfortably.

Tighten your pelvic floor muscles, hold for a count of three, then relax for a count of three.

Repeat 10 times.

Gradually increase the hold time to five seconds as your muscles get stronger.

2. Quick Flicks:

Tighten your pelvic floor muscles quickly and then relax immediately.

Repeat 10 times.

This exercise helps improve the quick response of your pelvic muscles.

3. Bridge with Pelvic Floor Activation:

  - Lie on your back with your knees bent and feet flat on the floor.

As you lift your hips into a bridge position, tighten your pelvic floor muscles.

Hold for a count of three, then lower your hips and relax your muscles.

Repeat 10 times.

4. Pelvic Tilts:

Lie on your back with your knees bent and feet flat on the floor.

Tighten your pelvic floor muscles and tilt your pelvis up slightly, flattening your back against the floor.

Hold for a count of three, then relax.

Repeat 10 times.

Consistency is key with these exercises. Aim to perform them daily, gradually increasing the number of repetitions and duration as your muscles get stronger. Remember, it's important to breathe normally and avoid holding your breath while performing these exercises.

PELVIC FLOOR EXERCISE TECHNIQUES

Maintaining a strong and healthy pelvic floor is essential for seniors to support bladder control, bowel function, and overall core stability. In this chapter, we'll explore various pelvic floor exercises, beginning with the renowned Kegel exercises, followed by additional movements that complement and enhance pelvic floor strength.

A. Kegel Exercises:

Kegel exercises, named after Dr. Arnold Kegel who developed them, are specifically designed to strengthen the pelvic floor muscles. These exercises are simple yet effective and can be done anywhere without any special equipment.

I. Step-by-Step Guide:

Step 1: Identify Your Pelvic Floor Muscles:

To begin, you need to locate your pelvic floor muscles. The easiest way to do this is to try stopping the flow of urine midstream. The muscles you use for this action are your pelvic floor muscles.

Step 2: Empty Your Bladder:

Before performing Kegel exercises, it's best to start with an empty bladder to avoid any discomfort.

Step 3: Find a Comfortable Position:

Sit or lie down in a comfortable position. Many people find it easiest to do Kegels while lying on their back.

Step 4: Contract the Muscles:

Tighten your pelvic floor muscles and hold the contraction for three to five seconds. You should feel a lifting sensation.

Step 5: Relax the Muscles:

Release the contraction and relax for an equal amount of time (three to five seconds).

Step 6: Repeat:

Perform 10 to 15 repetitions per session. Aim to do three sessions a day.

II. Variations and Intensity Levels:

Quick Flicks:

Quick flicks involve rapidly contracting and relaxing your pelvic floor muscles. This variation helps to improve the muscle's ability to respond quickly, which is useful for sudden movements like coughing or sneezing.

How to Perform Quick Flicks:

1. Tighten your pelvic floor muscles quickly and hold for one second.

2. Release immediately and relax for one second.

3. Repeat 10 to 15 times per session, up to three times daily.

Slow Holds:

Slow holds focus on building endurance in the pelvic floor muscles. This involves holding the contraction for a longer period.

How to Perform Slow Holds:

1. Tighten your pelvic floor muscles and hold for 10 seconds.

2. Slowly release and relax for 10 seconds.

3. Repeat five to 10 times per session, up to three times daily.

Increasing Intensity:

As your pelvic floor muscles become stronger, you can increase the intensity of your Kegel exercises by extending the duration of each hold, increasing the number of repetitions, or incorporating Kegels into other activities like standing or walking.

B. Beyond Kegels: Additional Exercises:

While Kegel exercises are excellent for targeting the pelvic floor, incorporating a variety of exercises can provide comprehensive benefits. Here are some additional exercises that support pelvic floor health.

I. Bridge:

The bridge exercise strengthens the glutes, lower back, and core muscles, which indirectly support the pelvic floor.

How to Perform the Bridge:

1. Lie on your back with your knees bent and feet flat on the floor, hip-width apart.

2. Place your arms at your sides with palms facing down.

3. Tighten your abdominal muscles and lift your hips off the ground, forming a straight line from your shoulders to your knees.

4. Squeeze your glutes and hold the position for three to five seconds.

5. Slowly lower your hips back to the starting position.

6. Repeat 10 to 15 times.

II. Squats:

Squats engage multiple muscle groups, including the pelvic floor, making them a powerful exercise for overall strength.

How to Perform Squats:

1. Stand with your feet shoulder-width apart and toes slightly turned out.

2. Lower your body by bending your knees and pushing your hips back, as if sitting in a chair.

3. Keep your back straight and your knees aligned over your toes.

4. Go as low as you can comfortably go, then push through your heels to return to the starting position.

5. Repeat 10 to 15 times.

III. Core Strengthening:

A strong core is essential for supporting the pelvic floor. Core exercises help stabilize the trunk and reduce strain on the pelvic area.

Plank:

How to Perform the Plank:

1. Lie face down on the floor.

2. Lift your body onto your toes and forearms, keeping your body in a straight line from head to heels.

3. Tighten your abdominal muscles and hold the position for 10 to 30 seconds.

4. Rest and repeat three to five times.

Bird Dog:

How to Perform the Bird Dog:

1. Start on your hands and knees, with your hands under your shoulders and knees under your hips.

2. Extend your right arm forward and your left leg back, keeping your body balanced and stable.

3. Hold for a few seconds, then return to the starting position.

4. Repeat with the left arm and right leg.

5. Perform 10 repetitions on each side.

Incorporating these exercises into your daily routine can significantly enhance the strength and function of your pelvic floor. Consistency is key, and over time, you'll likely notice improvements in both muscle control and overall pelvic health.

VAGINAL TRAINING AND DEVICES

Pelvic floor health is crucial for maintaining overall well-being, especially as we age. One effective way to strengthen the pelvic floor muscles is through vaginal training, which involves using various devices to enhance muscle tone and function. In this chapter, we will explore two main approaches: vaginal weight training and the use of biofeedback and electrical stimulation devices.

A. Vaginal Weight Training:

Vaginal weight training is a method that involves the use of specially designed weights to improve the strength and endurance of the pelvic floor muscles. This practice can help with issues such as urinary incontinence, pelvic organ prolapse, and overall pelvic health.

I. Types of Vaginal Weights:

1. Kegel Balls: Also known as Ben Wa balls, these are small, weighted balls that are inserted into the vagina. They come in various sizes and weights to suit different levels of training.

2. Vaginal Cones: These are cone-shaped devices that vary in weight. They are designed to be held in place by contracting the pelvic floor muscles.

3. Weighted Vaginal Eggs: Similar to Kegel balls, these are egg-shaped weights that are often made from materials like metal or jade. They provide a natural feel and come in different weights.

4. Progressive Weight Sets: These sets include multiple weights that allow users to gradually increase the resistance as their pelvic floor muscles strengthen.

II. Proper Usage and Benefits:

1. Proper Usage:

Choosing the Right Weight: Start with a lighter weight and gradually increase as your strength improves. It's important to listen to your body and not overexert yourself.

Insertion: Relax and gently insert the weight into the vagina, positioning it comfortably. Some find it helpful to use a bit of lubricant.

Training Routine: Contract and lift the pelvic floor muscles, holding the weight in place. Begin with short sessions, such as 5-10 minutes, and gradually increase the duration.

Consistency: For best results, perform these exercises regularly, aiming for at least a few times per week.

2. Benefits:

Strengthening Muscles: Regular use of vaginal weights can significantly strengthen the pelvic floor muscles, helping to alleviate symptoms of incontinence and prolapse.

Improved Control: Enhanced muscle tone can lead to better control over bladder and bowel movements.

Enhanced Sexual Function: Stronger pelvic floor muscles can increase sensitivity and improve sexual satisfaction.

Support for Pelvic Organs: Strengthening the pelvic floor provides better support for the bladder, uterus, and rectum, reducing the risk of prolapse.

B. Biofeedback and Electrical Stimulation:

Biofeedback and electrical stimulation are advanced techniques that can aid in pelvic floor training. These methods use devices to provide real-time feedback and stimulate muscle contractions, making exercises more effective.

I. How These Tools Work:

1. Biofeedback Devices:

Function: Biofeedback devices measure muscle activity and provide visual or auditory feedback. This helps users understand how effectively they are contracting their pelvic floor muscles.

Usage: A sensor is placed in the vagina or on the perineum, which detects muscle contractions. The device then provides feedback, allowing users to adjust their technique and improve muscle control.

2. Electrical Stimulation Devices:

Function: These devices use mild electrical currents to stimulate pelvic floor muscles, causing them to contract. This can be particularly helpful for individuals who have difficulty performing voluntary contractions.

Usage: A probe is inserted into the vagina, and the device delivers controlled electrical pulses. Users can adjust the intensity and frequency of the stimulation according to their comfort level.

II. Using Devices Safely and Effectively:

1. Safety Guidelines:

Consult a Healthcare Provider: Before starting any new training regimen, especially with electrical stimulation, consult a healthcare professional to ensure it's appropriate for your condition.

Follow Instructions: Carefully read and follow the manufacturer's instructions for each device to ensure safe and effective use.

Hygiene: Clean devices thoroughly before and after each use to prevent infections.

Avoid Overuse: Start with short sessions and gradually increase duration and intensity. Overuse can lead to muscle fatigue or injury.

2. Effective Usage:

Consistency: Regular use is key to seeing benefits. Aim to use these devices a few times per week, or as recommended by your healthcare provider.

Combine with Other Exercises: For optimal results, combine biofeedback and electrical stimulation with other pelvic floor exercises, such as Kegels.

Monitor Progress: Keep track of your progress and any changes in symptoms. This can help you and your healthcare provider adjust your training program as needed.

Vaginal training devices, when used correctly, can be powerful tools for enhancing pelvic floor strength and improving quality of life. Whether you opt for vaginal weights, biofeedback, or electrical stimulation, incorporating these methods into your routine can lead to significant benefits in pelvic health. Always remember to consult with healthcare professionals to tailor a program that best suits your individual needs and health status.

RELAXATION TECHNIQUES FOR PELVIC FLOOR HEALTH

Maintaining pelvic floor health involves more than just strengthening exercises. Relaxation is equally vital for a balanced and functional pelvic floor. In this chapter, we will explore the importance of relaxation, its role in balancing muscle strength, and how it helps reduce tension and pain. We will also introduce some effective relaxation exercises specifically designed to support pelvic floor health in seniors.

A. Importance of Relaxation:

Relaxation is often overlooked in the pursuit of physical fitness, but it is an essential component of a comprehensive approach to pelvic floor health. The muscles of the pelvic floor, like any other muscle group, need to be able to both contract and relax effectively. Failing to balance strength with relaxation can lead to muscle tension, discomfort, and even pain.

I. Balancing Muscle Strength with Relaxation:

The pelvic floor muscles support various bodily functions and contribute to core stability. While strengthening these muscles is important, it is equally crucial to allow them to relax. Overly tense muscles can become fatigued and less effective, potentially leading to problems such as urinary incontinence or pelvic pain. Relaxation helps maintain muscle elasticity, ensuring that the pelvic floor can function optimally.

A balanced approach to pelvic floor health involves alternating between exercises that strengthen and those that relax the muscles. This balance prevents muscle overuse and strain, promoting overall well-being and functionality.

II. Reducing Tension and Pain:

Chronic tension in the pelvic floor muscles can result in discomfort and pain, impacting daily activities and quality of life. Relaxation techniques can alleviate this tension, providing relief from symptoms and preventing further issues. By incorporating regular relaxation practices, seniors can manage and reduce pain associated with pelvic floor dysfunction.

Reducing tension in the pelvic floor not only helps in managing pain but also improves blood flow to the area, enhancing healing and overall muscle health. This holistic approach can significantly improve the quality of life for seniors.

B. Relaxation Exercises:

There are several relaxation exercises that can benefit the pelvic floor. These techniques can be easily incorporated into a daily routine and can complement other pelvic floor exercises. Below are three effective relaxation exercises specifically designed for pelvic floor health.

I. Deep Breathing:

Deep breathing is a simple yet powerful relaxation technique that can have a profound effect on the pelvic floor. This exercise promotes relaxation by encouraging the muscles to release tension and allows for better oxygen flow throughout the body.

To practice deep breathing:

1. Find a comfortable position: Sit or lie down in a relaxed position, ensuring that your body is supported.

2. Inhale deeply: Breathe in slowly through your nose, allowing your abdomen to rise as your lungs fill with air.

3. Exhale slowly: Breathe out gently through your mouth, letting your abdomen fall.

4. Focus on the breath: Concentrate on the rhythm of your breathing, allowing each breath to become slower and deeper.

Repeat this process for several minutes, focusing on the sensation of relaxation spreading through your pelvic floor with each exhale.

II. Progressive Muscle Relaxation:

Progressive muscle relaxation (PMR) is a technique that involves tensing and then relaxing different muscle groups in the body. This method helps in identifying and releasing tension in the pelvic floor.

To practice PMR:

1. Find a quiet space: Sit or lie down in a comfortable position.

2. Tense a muscle group: Start with your feet and work your way up. Tense each muscle group for a few seconds.

3. Release the tension: Gradually release the tension and focus on the feeling of relaxation that follows.

4. Progress to the next group: Move to the next muscle group and repeat the process.

When you reach the pelvic floor, gently tighten the muscles as if you are trying to stop the flow of urine, hold for a few seconds, then slowly release and focus on the relaxation.

III. Pelvic Floor Drops:

Pelvic floor drops are a specific relaxation exercise designed to help the pelvic floor muscles release and lengthen. This exercise counterbalances the contractions performed during strengthening exercises.

To practice pelvic floor drops:

1. Find a comfortable position:MN Sit or lie down in a position that allows you to focus on your pelvic area.

2. Identify your pelvic floor muscles: Visualize the muscles that you use to stop the flow of urine.

3. Relax the muscles: Take a deep breath in, and as you exhale, consciously relax and

"drop" the pelvic floor muscles, allowing them to release any tension.

4. Repeat the process: Perform this exercise for a few minutes, ensuring that you focus on the sensation of the muscles dropping and relaxing.

By incorporating these relaxation exercises into your routine, you can enhance the overall health and functionality of your pelvic floor. Remember, the goal is to achieve a balance between strength and relaxation, promoting a pain-free and well-functioning pelvic floor.

In the next chapter, we will delve into specific strengthening exercises tailored for seniors, providing a comprehensive approach to maintaining pelvic floor health. Balancing these with the relaxation techniques covered in this chapter will ensure a holistic and effective pelvic floor exercise regimen.

ADDRESSING INCONTINENCE

A. Understanding Incontinence:

Incontinence is a condition that affects many seniors, significantly impacting their daily lives and overall well-being. To effectively address this issue, it is essential to understand its causes, types, and the profound influence it has on quality of life.

I. Causes and Types:

1. Causes of Incontinence:

Incontinence can result from various factors, including:

Weak Pelvic Floor Muscles: As we age, the muscles supporting the bladder and urethra can weaken, leading to incontinence.

Neurological Disorders: Conditions like Parkinson's disease, multiple sclerosis, and stroke can disrupt the nerve signals involved in bladder control.

Medications: Some medications, including diuretics, can increase urine production or interfere with bladder control.

Chronic Conditions: Diabetes, obesity, and chronic cough from smoking can contribute to incontinence.

Hormonal Changes: Post-menopausal women often experience a decrease in estrogen levels, which can weaken the urethral tissue and lead to incontinence.

2. Types of Incontinence:

Understanding the different types of incontinence is crucial for selecting the appropriate exercises and treatments:

Stress Incontinence: This occurs when physical activities such as coughing, sneezing, laughing, or exercising put pressure on the bladder, leading to leakage. It is often due to weakened pelvic floor muscles.

Urge Incontinence: Also known as overactive bladder, this type involves a sudden, intense urge to urinate, followed by involuntary leakage. It can result from bladder muscle spasms or nerve damage.

Mixed Incontinence: This type is a combination of stress and urge incontinence, where individuals experience symptoms of both.

Overflow Incontinence: This occurs when the bladder cannot empty completely, leading to overflow and leakage. It is often associated with conditions that obstruct the bladder outlet or affect bladder contractility.

Functional Incontinence: This type is related to physical or cognitive impairments that prevent a person from reaching the bathroom in time, despite having normal bladder control.

II. Impact on Quality of Life:

Incontinence can profoundly affect a senior's quality of life, leading to:

Emotional Distress: Feelings of embarrassment, shame, and anxiety are common, as individuals may fear public leakage or odor.

Social Isolation: Many seniors may withdraw from social activities, leading to loneliness and depression.

Sleep Disruption: Nocturia (frequent nighttime urination) can disrupt sleep patterns, causing fatigue and affecting overall health.

Physical Health Issues: Constant moisture from urine can lead to skin infections and irritation.

Financial Burden: The cost of incontinence products, medications, and treatments can be substantial.

Recognizing the impact of incontinence on quality of life underscores the importance of effective management strategies, including pelvic floor exercises.

B. Exercise Protocols for Incontinence:

Pelvic floor exercises can be highly effective in managing incontinence, particularly stress and urge incontinence. Here, we outline specific exercise protocols tailored to each type.

I. Specific Exercises for Stress Incontinence:

Stress incontinence can be improved by strengthening the pelvic floor muscles. The following exercises are recommended:

1. Kegel Exercises:

Identify the Pelvic Floor Muscles: The first step is to locate the correct muscles by trying to stop urination midstream. Once identified, these are the muscles you will be exercising.

Performing Kegels: Contract the pelvic floor muscles, hold for 3-5 seconds, and then relax for the same amount of time. Gradually increase the hold time to 10 seconds as strength improves.

Repetitions: Aim for at least three sets of 10-15 repetitions daily.

2. Bridge Exercise:

Starting Position: Lie on your back with knees bent and feet flat on the floor, hip-width apart.

Execution: Tighten your pelvic floor muscles and lift your hips towards the ceiling, forming a straight line from knees to shoulders. Hold for 3-5 seconds and then lower your hips back down.

Repetitions: Perform 10-15 repetitions, three times a day.

3. Wall Squats:

Starting Position: Stand with your back against a wall and feet shoulder-width apart.

Execution: Tighten your pelvic floor muscles, slide down the wall into a squat position, and hold for 5 seconds. Then, slowly return to the starting position.

Repetitions: Perform 10 repetitions, two to three times daily.

II. Managing Urge Incontinence with Relaxation:

Urge incontinence can often be managed through relaxation techniques aimed at calming the bladder and reducing the urge to urinate.

1. Bladder Training:

Scheduled Voiding: Establish a regular schedule for bathroom visits, starting with every two hours. Gradually increase the interval between visits by 15 minutes each week until reaching a 3-4 hour interval.

Delay Tactics: When the urge strikes, try to delay urination by using relaxation techniques such as deep breathing or pelvic floor contractions (quick Kegels).

2. Deep Breathing and Meditation:

Deep Breathing: Practice slow, deep breathing to help calm the bladder muscles. Inhale deeply through the nose, hold for a few seconds, and then exhale slowly through the mouth.

Meditation: Incorporate mindfulness meditation to reduce stress and anxiety, which can exacerbate urge incontinence. Focus on relaxing the entire body, especially the pelvic area.

3. Toe Tapping:

Starting Position: Sit comfortably with your feet flat on the floor.

Execution: When you feel the urge to urinate, tap your toes rapidly for a few seconds. This can help distract the brain and reduce the intensity of the urge.

Repetitions: Repeat as necessary until the urge diminishes.

MANAGING CONSTIPATION

Constipation is a common concern among seniors, often resulting from a combination of factors including decreased physical activity, dietary changes, medications, and the natural aging process. In this chapter, we will delve into how the pelvic floor influences bowel function and explore effective strategies and exercises to manage and alleviate constipation.

A. The Pelvic Floor and Bowel Function:

I. How the Pelvic Floor Affects Constipation:

The pelvic floor muscles play a crucial role in bowel function. These muscles form a supportive sling at the base of the pelvis, controlling the release of stool from the rectum. When the pelvic floor muscles are weakened or not functioning correctly, it can lead to difficulties with bowel movements, contributing to constipation.

1. Pelvic Floor Dysfunction: When the pelvic floor muscles are too tight or too weak, it can hinder the ability to effectively push stool out of the rectum. Tight muscles may lead to incomplete evacuation, while weak muscles can cause a lack of coordination necessary for bowel movements.

2. Rectal Prolapse: In severe cases of pelvic floor dysfunction, rectal prolapse may occur, where the rectum protrudes through the anus. This condition can complicate bowel movements and exacerbate constipation.

3. Coordination Issues: Proper coordination of the pelvic floor muscles is essential for bowel movements. When these muscles do not work in harmony, it can lead to difficulty in stool passage and increased straining, further contributing to constipation.

II. Lifestyle and Dietary Adjustments:

In addition to understanding the role of the pelvic floor, making certain lifestyle and dietary adjustments can significantly alleviate constipation.

1. Hydration: Staying well-hydrated is crucial for maintaining soft stools and promoting regular bowel movements. Seniors should aim to drink plenty of water throughout the day.

2. Dietary Fiber: A diet rich in fiber can help regulate bowel movements. Incorporating whole grains, fruits, vegetables, and legumes into daily meals can enhance stool bulk and ease its passage.

3. Regular Physical Activity: Engaging in regular exercise, such as walking, swimming, or gentle yoga, can stimulate bowel function and reduce the incidence of constipation.

4. Routine: Establishing a regular bowel routine by trying to go to the bathroom at the

same time each day can help train the body and reduce episodes of constipation.

5. Mindful Eating: Eating meals at regular intervals and chewing food thoroughly can aid digestion and promote more regular bowel movements.

B. Exercises to Relieve Constipation:

Exercise can be an effective way to alleviate constipation by improving bowel function and strengthening the pelvic floor muscles.

I. Techniques to Promote Regular Bowel Movements:

1. Pelvic Floor Relaxation: Learning to relax the pelvic floor muscles during bowel movements can help reduce straining. Techniques such as deep breathing and gentle abdominal massage can encourage relaxation.

2.Squatting Position: Adopting a squatting position can help straighten the rectum and facilitate easier bowel movements. Using a footstool to elevate the feet while sitting on the toilet can mimic the squatting position.

3. Pelvic Tilts: Performing pelvic tilts can help stimulate bowel movements. Lie on your back with knees bent and feet flat on the floor. Tilt your pelvis upwards and hold for a few seconds before lowering back down. Repeat several times.

4. Abdominal Massages: Gentle abdominal massages can help stimulate the intestines and promote bowel movements. Using circular motions, massage the abdomen starting from the lower right side, moving up to the rib cage, across to the left side, and down towards the lower left abdomen.

II. Relaxation Strategies for Bowel Health:

1. Deep Breathing Exercises: Deep breathing can help relax the pelvic floor muscles and

reduce stress, which can contribute to constipation. Practice slow, deep breaths in through the nose and out through the mouth, focusing on relaxing the abdominal muscles.

2. Progressive Muscle Relaxation: This technique involves tensing and then relaxing different muscle groups in the body, including the pelvic floor. It can help increase awareness of muscle tension and promote relaxation.

3. Mindfulness Meditation: Practicing mindfulness meditation can reduce stress and improve overall digestive health. Focus on deep breathing and being present in the moment, which can help relax the body and support regular bowel function.

4. Visualization Techniques: Visualizing the process of a smooth, effortless bowel movement can help mentally prepare the body for successful elimination. Close your eyes and imagine a relaxed, easy passage of stool.

HEALING PELVIC PAIN

A. Causes of Pelvic Pain:

I. Common Sources and Symptoms:

Pelvic pain can manifest for a multitude of reasons, often leading to discomfort and disruption in daily life for seniors. Understanding the origins and identifying symptoms are crucial steps towards effective management. Among the common sources of pelvic pain are:

1. Musculoskeletal Issues: Conditions such as arthritis, muscle strains, or ligament sprains can lead to pelvic discomfort. Seniors, due to age-related changes in bone density and muscle strength, are particularly susceptible to these issues.

2. Pelvic Organ Disorders: Conditions affecting the bladder, uterus, ovaries, or prostate can cause pelvic pain. Examples include urinary tract infections (UTIs), pelvic

inflammatory disease (PID), or benign prostatic hyperplasia (BPH).

3. Nerve Disorders: Nerve damage or irritation, such as from sciatica or pudendal neuralgia, can result in pelvic pain. These conditions may cause sensations of tingling, burning, or numbness in the pelvic region.

4. Gastrointestinal Disorders: Digestive issues like irritable bowel syndrome (IBS), constipation, or diverticulitis can also manifest with pelvic pain, often due to referred pain from the intestines.

Recognizing the symptoms associated with these sources is essential for accurate diagnosis and targeted treatment. Symptoms may include persistent or intermittent pain in the pelvic area, lower back pain, urinary urgency or frequency, bowel irregularities, sexual dysfunction, or discomfort during sitting or movement.

II. The Role of Muscle Tension and Spasms:

Muscle tension and spasms play a significant role in pelvic pain, often exacerbating discomfort and contributing to its chronicity. Seniors, particularly those with sedentary lifestyles or underlying health conditions, are prone to muscle tightness and imbalances in the pelvic floor muscles.

1. Pelvic Floor Dysfunction: Dysfunction in the pelvic floor muscles, characterized by hypertonicity or weakness, can lead to pelvic pain. Hypertonic muscles are overly tense and contracted, causing pain and dysfunction, while weak muscles may fail to provide adequate support, leading to instability and discomfort.

2. Trigger Points: Trigger points, or localized areas of muscle tightness and tenderness, can develop in the pelvic floor muscles due to various factors such as overuse, poor posture, or stress. These trigger points can refer pain to other areas of the body, exacerbating pelvic discomfort.

3. Inflammation and Irritation: Chronic tension in the pelvic floor muscles can lead to inflammation and irritation of surrounding tissues, further perpetuating the cycle of pain. Psychological factors such as anxiety or depression can also contribute to muscle tension and amplify pelvic pain symptoms.

Understanding the interplay between muscle tension, spasms, and pelvic pain is crucial for developing effective treatment strategies that target the root cause of the discomfort.

B. Exercise and Relaxation for Pain Relief:

I. Tailored Exercises for Pain Management:

Exercise plays a pivotal role in managing pelvic pain by addressing muscle imbalances, improving flexibility, and enhancing overall pelvic floor function. Tailored exercises designed specifically for seniors can help alleviate pain and promote pelvic health.

1. Pelvic Floor Muscle Exercises (Kegels): Kegel exercises are designed to strengthen the pelvic floor muscles, improving their tone and endurance. Seniors can benefit from incorporating Kegels into their daily routine to enhance bladder and bowel control, reduce pelvic pain, and support pelvic organ function.

2. Stretching and Mobility Exercises: Gentle stretching exercises targeting the pelvic floor muscles, hip flexors, and lower back can help alleviate muscle tension and improve flexibility. Incorporating movements such as pelvic tilts, hip circles, and gentle yoga poses can promote relaxation and reduce pelvic discomfort.

II. Integrating Relaxation to Ease Discomfort:

In addition to targeted exercises, relaxation techniques are essential for managing pelvic pain and reducing muscle tension. Seniors can explore various relaxation strategies to complement their exercise routine and promote overall well-being.

1. Deep Breathing: Deep breathing exercises, such as diaphragmatic breathing or progressive muscle relaxation, can help seniors release tension in the pelvic floor muscles and promote relaxation throughout the body.

2. Mind-Body Practices: Mindfulness meditation, guided imagery, or tai chi can help seniors cultivate awareness of bodily sensations, reduce stress, and alleviate pelvic pain. These mind-body practices encourage relaxation and foster a sense of calm amidst discomfort.

3. Warm Baths or Heat Therapy: Soaking in a warm bath or applying heat packs to the pelvic area can provide immediate relief from pelvic pain by relaxing tense muscles and increasing blood flow to the area.

CREATING A SUSTAINABLE EXERCISE ROUTINE

A. Developing a Consistent Practice:

I. Setting Realistic Goals:

In the journey to improve pelvic floor health, setting realistic goals is paramount. Seniors embarking on pelvic floor exercises must understand that progress may not always be linear, and that's perfectly normal. Rather than aiming for drastic changes overnight, it's essential to set achievable milestones that align with individual capabilities and health conditions.

When setting goals, consider factors such as current fitness level, medical history, and lifestyle. For instance, if a senior is just starting out with pelvic floor exercises, a realistic goal could be to perform basic exercises for a certain duration each day, gradually increasing intensity and duration as strength improves.

Remember, the key is to set goals that are challenging yet attainable. This helps maintain motivation and prevents discouragement. Celebrate each milestone achieved, whether it's holding a contraction for a few seconds longer or experiencing fewer episodes of urinary incontinence. Every step forward, no matter how small, is a victory in the journey toward better pelvic floor health.

II. Tracking Progress:

Tracking progress is essential for staying motivated and making informed adjustments to your exercise routine. By keeping a record of your pelvic floor exercises, you can identify patterns, track improvements, and adjust your goals accordingly.

There are various ways to track progress, depending on personal preference and convenience. Some seniors may prefer using a traditional pen-and-paper journal to log their exercises, noting down the type of exercises performed, duration, and any observations or challenges encountered. Others may opt for digital apps or devices that offer features such as exercise reminders, progress tracking, and even biofeedback.

Regardless of the method chosen, consistency is key. Make it a habit to review your progress regularly, perhaps at the end of each week or month. Celebrate achievements, no matter how small, and use setbacks as learning opportunities to refine your approach.

B. Incorporating Exercises into Daily Life:

I. Simple Exercises during Daily Activities:

Incorporating pelvic floor exercises into daily life doesn't always require dedicated workout sessions. Many exercises can be seamlessly integrated into everyday activities, making pelvic floor health a natural part of daily routine.

For example, practicing kegel exercises while sitting or standing in line, waiting for the kettle to boil, or during commercial breaks while watching television can be effective ways to sneak in extra repetitions throughout the day. These discreet exercises not only contribute to strengthening the pelvic floor muscles but also serve as gentle reminders to prioritize pelvic floor health in everyday life.

II. Making Pelvic Floor Health a Lifelong Habit:

Pelvic floor health is not a short-term endeavor but a lifelong commitment. As seniors, it's important to recognize the significance of maintaining pelvic floor strength and function as part of overall health and well-being.

To make pelvic floor health a lifelong habit, cultivate mindfulness and awareness of your body's needs. Listen to your body and adjust your exercise routine accordingly, adapting to changes in physical condition and lifestyle. Stay informed about pelvic floor health by seeking reliable sources of information and consulting healthcare professionals as needed.

Additionally, foster a supportive environment by surrounding yourself with peers who share similar goals and experiences. Joining pelvic floor exercise classes or support groups can provide valuable encouragement, accountability, and camaraderie on the journey toward sustained pelvic floor health.

By integrating pelvic floor exercises into daily life and nurturing a mindset of lifelong commitment, seniors can empower themselves to maintain optimal pelvic floor health well into their golden years.

CASE STUDIES AND SUCCESS STORIES

In this chapter, we delve into the real-life experiences of seniors who have embraced pelvic floor exercises and witnessed remarkable transformations in their health and well-being. Through their testimonials and stories, we gain insights into the challenges they faced and the triumphs they achieved.

I. Testimonials from Seniors Who Benefited from Exercises:

Martha's Story: Reclaiming Confidence and Control:

At 73, Martha found herself struggling with urinary incontinence, a common issue among seniors that can severely impact one's quality of life. Embarrassed and frustrated, Martha was hesitant to seek help until she stumbled upon pelvic floor exercises.

"After just a few weeks of consistently practicing pelvic floor exercises, I noticed a significant improvement," Martha recounts. "Not only did my leakage decrease, but I also regained control over my bladder. I feel more confident now, knowing that I'm not limited by my condition."

Martha's story reflects the transformative power of pelvic floor exercises in addressing urinary incontinence, restoring her confidence, and enhancing her overall well-being.

Robert's Journey: Finding Relief from Chronic Pain:

For years, 68-year-old Robert battled with chronic pelvic pain, a debilitating condition that greatly hindered his daily activities. Despite trying various treatments, relief seemed elusive until he discovered the therapeutic benefits of pelvic floor exercises.

"Initially, I was skeptical, but I was desperate for relief," Robert shares. "To my surprise, as I committed to a regimen of pelvic floor exercises recommended by my physiotherapist, I experienced gradual but significant reduction in my pain levels. It's been a game-changer for me."

Robert's testimonial underscores the effectiveness of pelvic floor exercises in alleviating chronic pelvic pain, offering hope and relief to seniors grappling with similar challenges.

II. Overcoming Challenges and Achieving Results:

Sarah's Struggle: Overcoming Skepticism and Inertia:

At 65, Sarah was skeptical about the efficacy of pelvic floor exercises in addressing her pelvic organ prolapse, a condition that caused discomfort and distress. However, with encouragement from her healthcare provider,

Sarah embarked on a journey of perseverance and determination.

"It wasn't easy at first," Sarah admits. "I struggled to stay consistent with the exercises, and doubts crept in. But as I persisted, I began to notice subtle improvements. My symptoms diminished, and I felt stronger and more in control."

Sarah's story exemplifies the importance of overcoming skepticism and inertia, highlighting the transformative impact of persistence and commitment to pelvic floor exercises.

John's Triumph: Regaining Independence and Mobility

:Following prostate surgery at the age of 70, John faced challenges with urinary incontinence and diminished mobility, threatening his independence. Determined to reclaim his autonomy, John embraced pelvic floor exercises as part of his rehabilitation journey.

"Initially, it was tough," John recalls. "But with guidance from my healthcare team and consistent effort, I gradually regained control over my bladder and strengthened my pelvic muscles. Now, I can enjoy activities I once took for granted, like hiking and gardening, with confidence."

John's journey serves as a testament to the transformative power of pelvic floor exercises in restoring independence, mobility, and quality of life for seniors navigating post-surgery challenges.

Through these case studies and success stories, we witness the profound impact of pelvic floor exercises in empowering seniors to overcome adversity, reclaim their health, and embrace life with renewed vitality and confidence.

CONCLUSION

In concluding our journey through "Pelvic Floor Exercises for Seniors," it is imperative to recap the key points that underscore the transformative potential of pelvic floor exercises and the encouragement to maintain a proactive approach towards pelvic health.

I. The transformative potential of pelvic floor exercises:

Throughout this book, we have delved into the profound impact that pelvic floor exercises can have on seniors' overall well-being. From alleviating symptoms of urinary incontinence and pelvic organ prolapse to enhancing sexual function and promoting better posture and stability, the benefits are undeniable. Through consistent and targeted exercise, seniors can regain control over their pelvic muscles, leading to improved confidence, comfort, and quality of life. By prioritizing pelvic floor health, individuals can embrace aging with strength and vitality, knowing that they hold the power to positively influence their own physical and emotional wellness.

II. Encouragement to maintain a proactive approach:

As we conclude our exploration, let us emphasize the importance of maintaining a proactive approach to pelvic floor health. Consistency is key when it comes to exercise, and integrating pelvic floor exercises into daily routines can yield significant long-term benefits. Let us not wait for symptoms to escalate before taking action; instead, let us embrace a proactive mindset, prioritizing preventive measures and self-care practices. By nurturing our pelvic floor health today, we lay the foundation for a vibrant and fulfilling future, free from the limitations often associated with aging.

Moreover, for those seeking additional support and guidance on their pelvic floor journey, a wealth of resources is available:

B. Resources for Further Support:

I. Additional reading and exercises:

Explore further by delving into additional reading materials and exercises tailored to pelvic floor health. Numerous books, articles, and online resources offer comprehensive information and step-by-step guides to help individuals deepen their understanding and refine their pelvic floor exercise routines.

II. Professional organizations and support groups:

Connect with professional organizations and support groups dedicated to pelvic floor health. These communities provide valuable resources, expert guidance, and a supportive network of individuals sharing similar experiences. Whether seeking advice from healthcare professionals or camaraderie from peers, these organizations offer a holistic approach to pelvic floor wellness.

"Pelvic Floor Exercises for Seniors" serves as a roadmap towards improved pelvic health and overall well-being. By embracing the transformative potential of pelvic floor exercises and maintaining a proactive approach, seniors can embark on a journey of empowerment, reclaiming control over their bodies and embracing the fullness of life's possibilities. Let us step forward with confidence, knowing that with dedication and determination, pelvic floor health is within reach for every individual, regardless of age or circumstance.

THE END

www.ingramcontent.com/pod-product-compliance
Lightning Source LLC
Chambersburg PA
CBHW052336220526
45472CB00001B/450